THE BIRTH CONTROL PILL

Taking Control of Your Reproductive Health

By

Dr. Elizabeth M. Harris

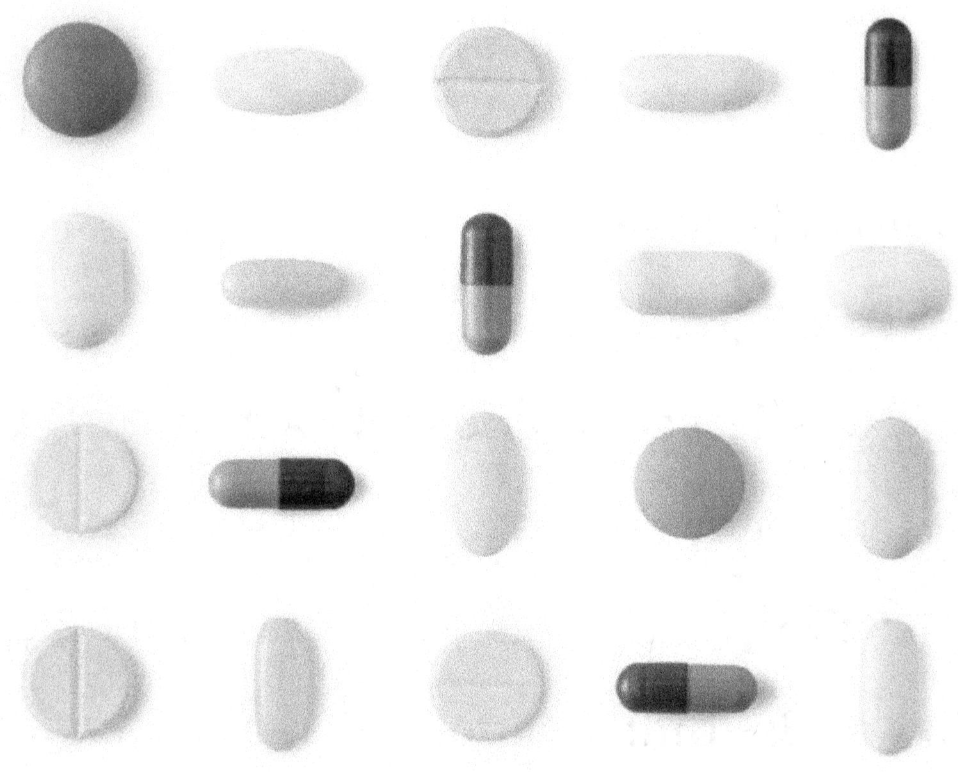

INTRODUCTION

As a woman, I understand the importance of contraception in planning and controlling my reproductive health. One of the most popular forms of birth control is the pill, and I've had my fair share of experiences with it. In this book, I will share my personal experiences with the birth control pill, from the initial decision to start using it, to the pros and cons I've encountered along the way.

The decision to start using birth control pills wasn't an easy one for me. As a teenager, I had heard stories from friends about the negative side effects of hormonal birth control, which left me feeling hesitant. However, I eventually decided to take the plunge after doing my own research and discussing my options with my doctor. After all, I wanted to take control of my reproductive health and the pill seemed like the best option for me at the time.

The first few months on the pill were a bit of an adjustment. I experienced some mild side effects like nausea and headaches, but these eventually subsided. However, what stood out to me the most was the peace of mind it gave me. Knowing that I was taking active steps to prevent pregnancy allowed me to relax and focus on other areas of my life.

Over the years, I've had a few different types of birth control pills, and each one has had its own set of pros and cons. For example, some pills caused my periods to become lighter and shorter, which was a welcomed change. However, other pills caused my periods to become irregular or caused breakthrough bleeding, which was frustrating. Some pills have also caused me to experience mood changes and a decreased sex drive, while others have had no effect on my mood or libido.

Despite these challenges, I still consider the birth control pill to be a valuable tool in managing my reproductive health. It has allowed me to plan and control my family size, given me the freedom to enjoy my sexuality without fear of unintended pregnancy, and provided a level of convenience that fits my lifestyle.

One of the most significant benefits of the birth control pill is its effectiveness in preventing pregnancy. When used correctly, it has a very high success rate, making it an excellent option for women who don't want to get pregnant. It also provides a level of privacy and control, as women can take it discreetly and without the involvement of a partner.

Another benefit is the flexibility it provides. With many different types of pills available, women can choose one that best suits their needs and preferences. For example, some pills contain a combination of hormones, while others only contain one hormone. Women can also choose pills that allow them to have fewer periods or no periods at all.

Of course, like any medication, birth control pills do have some risks and side effects. Women who smoke, are overweight, or have a history of blood clots or stroke may not be good candidates for hormonal birth control. The pill can also increase the risk of certain cancers and can cause other health issues, such as high blood pressure, gallbladder disease, and liver tumors.

My experience with the birth control pill has been largely positive. It has allowed me to take control of my reproductive health, given me the freedom to enjoy my sexuality, and provided a level of convenience that fits my lifestyle. While it's not perfect and has its own set of risks and side effects,

I believe it's an important tool for women to consider when making decisions about their reproductive health. Ultimately, the decision to use birth control is a personal one, and each woman should weigh the pros and cons and make the best decision for herself.

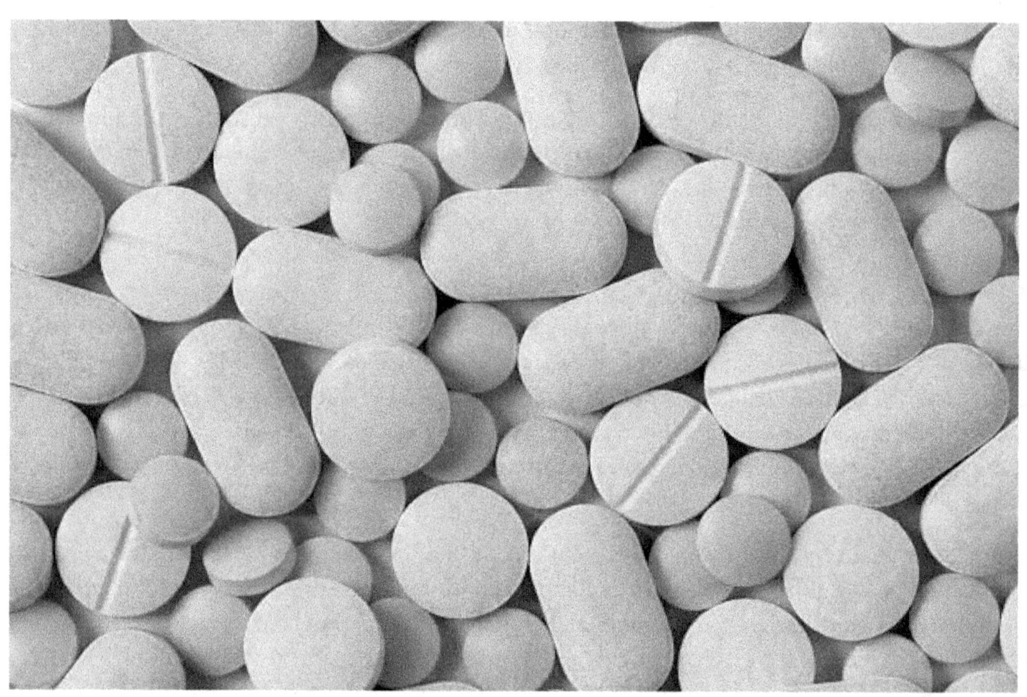

CHAPTER 1

Brief history of birth control

The history of birth control is lengthy and complicated, spanning thousands of years and many different civilizations. This is a more detailed account of the history of birth control.

Ancient civilizations: Many birth control techniques, including herbs and plants, have been employed by cultures across the globe for thousands of years. In ancient Egypt, women used a combination of crocodile dung and honey as a vaginal suppository to prevent conception. In ancient Greece, women utilized a vaginal barrier composed of olive oil-soaked wool. Other means of birth control used in ancient times included animal skins, dried camel dung, and sea sponges.

Early modern era: In the 16th century, condoms made of animal intestines started to be used in Europe to prevent pregnancy and protect against sexually transmitted illnesses. In the 19th century, introducing rubber condoms made them more readily accessible.

19th century: In the mid-19th century, the Comstock Laws were created in the United States, outlawing the spread of birth control knowledge and supplies. In 1873, the US Congress approved the Comstock Act, which prohibited the dissemination of contraceptive information over the mail.

20th century: In the early 20th century, the birth control movement gained steam in the United States and Europe. Women's rights campaigners like Margaret Sanger and Emma Goldman pushed to improve access to birth control and family planning services. In 1916, Sanger launched the first birth control clinic in the United States, which was shut down by authorities, and Sanger was jailed for breaking the Comstock Laws. In 1921, Sanger started the American Birth Control League (later renamed Planned Parenthood).

The 1920s-1930s: In the 1920s and 1930s, the diaphragm and other kinds of barrier techniques of birth control were increasingly commonly employed in the United States and Europe. In 1930, the birth control pill was invented by scientist Gregory Pincus, but it would take many more decades before it was widely marketed.

The 1940s-1950s: During World War II, the US military offered birth control to servicewomen. In the 1950s, the US Food and Drug Administration allowed using the diaphragm and other barrier techniques for birth control.

The 1960s: The development of the birth control pill in 1960 revolutionized contraception by providing a highly effective and easy means of birth control. The medicine swiftly became the most common type of birth control among women in the United States. In 1965, the Supreme Court threw down the restriction on birth control for married couples in the case of Griswold v. Connecticut.

The 1970s: The women's liberation movement of the 1970s drew heightened focus on concerns relating to reproductive health and access to birth control. In 1972, the Supreme Court determined in the case of Eisenstadt v. Baird that unmarried persons had the right to obtain contraceptives. In 1973, the Supreme Court legalized abortion in the historic decision of Roe v. Wade.

The 1980s-1990s: In the 1980s and 1990s, new kinds of hormonal birth control, such as the Depo-Provera injection and the Norplant implant, were available. In 1990, the FDA authorized the first emergency contraceptive pill (Plan B).

21st century: Currently, a broad range of birth control techniques are accessible, including hormonal and non-hormonal choices, as well as long-acting reversible contraception such as intrauterine devices (IUDs) and implants. In 2010, the Affordable Care

Definition of birth control

Birth control refers to procedures and equipment that are used to prevent conception. The use of birth control is meant to give individuals control over their reproductive health and enable them to plan and space out their pregnancies according to their choices and life circumstances.

There are many various forms of birth control available, including hormonal techniques such as birth control pills, patches, injections, and vaginal rings, as well as non-hormonal methods such as barrier methods like condoms, diaphragms, cervical caps, and spermicides. Long-acting reversible contraception (LARC), such as intrauterine devices (IUDs) and implants, are also available, as are sterilization treatments, including tubal ligation (female sterilization) and vasectomy (male sterilization).

The choice of birth control technique will rely on individual requirements, preferences, and medical factors. Some methods require a prescription from a healthcare physician, while others may be acquired over the counter. Using birth control regularly and appropriately is crucial to avoid unplanned births.

In addition to avoiding conception, birth control may have additional health advantages. For example, hormonal birth control may help regulate menstrual periods, minimize menstrual cramps, and improve acne. Certain forms of birth control may also lessen the risk of some kinds of cancer, such as ovarian and endometrial cancer.

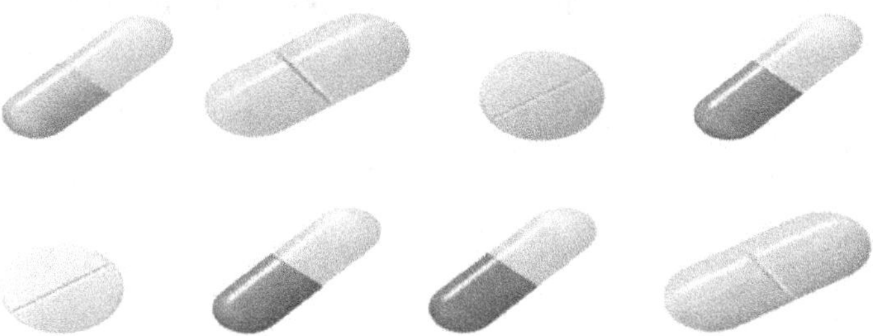

Importance of birth control

The value of birth control cannot be emphasized. These are some of the primary reasons why birth control is essential:

1. **Preventing unplanned pregnancies:** Birth control helps individuals to avoid unexpected births, which may have enormous societal, economic, and personal implications. Unintended pregnancies might result in women dropping out of school or job, limiting their professional progress and lowering their earning potential. They may also strain relationships and have a bad influence on mental health.

2. **Managing family size:** Birth control helps individuals plan and spread out their pregnancies according to their choices and living circumstances. This may assist in guaranteeing that children are born into families who are emotionally and financially equipped to care for them.

3. **Lowering maternal and infant mortality:** Unintended pregnancies are related to higher maternal and newborn mortality rates. Birth control may help reduce these rates by enabling women to spread out their pregnancies and better prepare for motherhood.

4. **Handling medical disorders:** Birth control may be used to address medical conditions such as endometriosis, polycystic ovarian syndrome (PCOS), and excessive menstrual flow. Hormonal birth control may also help regulate menstrual cycles and alleviate the symptoms of premenstrual syndrome (PMS).

5. **Supporting gender equality:** Access to birth control may assist in promoting gender equality by providing women control over their reproductive health and enabling them to pursue education and professional possibilities.

6. **Enhancing financial results:** Access to birth control has improved economic outcomes for people and communities. When individuals have control over their reproductive health, they can better plan for their futures, seek educational and job opportunities, and contribute to the economy.

7. **Preventing the transmission of sexually transmitted diseases (STIs):** Barrier birth control methods, such as condoms, may help decrease the spread of STIs. Utilizing a barrier technique with other birth control may protect against unwanted pregnancy and STIs.

8. **Enhancing overall health outcomes:** Birth control has been linked to improved health outcomes for people and communities. For example, access to birth control has been linked with decreased rates of HIV transmission, fewer unwanted pregnancies and abortions, and better mother and child health outcomes.

9. **Offering reproductive autonomy:** Access to birth control allows people to make educated decisions about their reproductive health and exercise control over their bodies. This may foster empowerment and independence, which is beneficial for general well-being.

10. **Safeguarding the environment:** Unplanned pregnancies may harm the environment by contributing to overpopulation and resource depletion. Birth control promotes sustainability and protects the earth by reducing unexpected births.

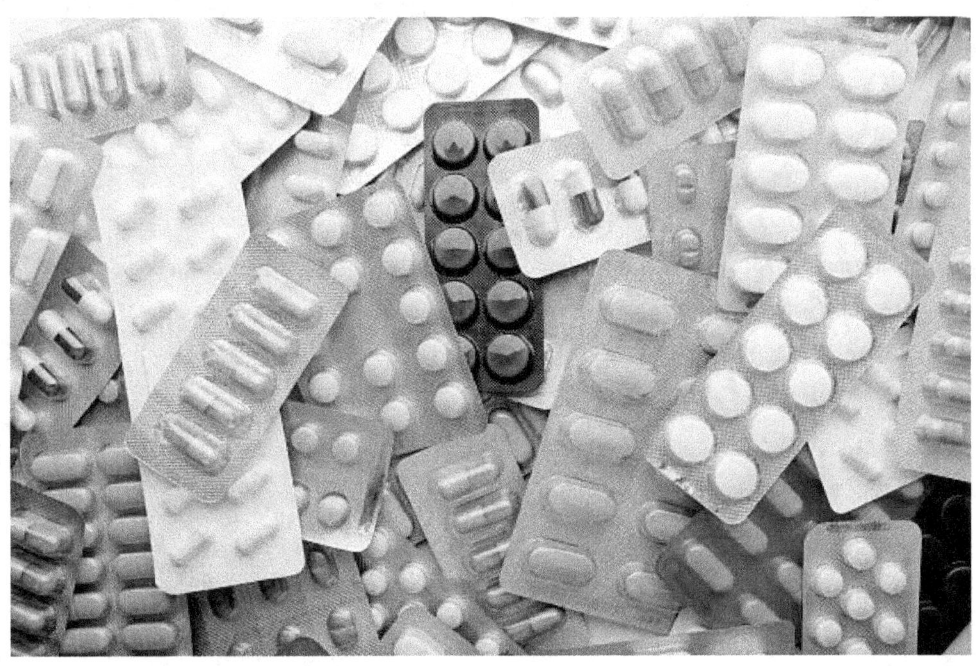

CHAPTER 2

Various birth control methods are available, each with pros and downsides. Following are some of the most prevalent forms of birth control:

Hormonal techniques

Hormonal methods of birth control involve hormones, often estrogen and progestin, to prevent pregnancy. These treatments operate by inhibiting ovulation, which is the release of an egg from the ovaries. Without ovulation, there is no egg for the sperm to fertilize, and pregnancy cannot occur.

Following are some of the most frequent hormonal methods of birth control

1. **Birth control pill:** The birth control pill is a daily tablet that includes hormones, either a mix of estrogen and progestin or only progestin. When used correctly, the medicine is up to 99% effective in preventing pregnancy. Many kinds of birth control pills are available, with differing levels of hormones and dose regimens.
2. **Patch:** The birth control patch is a little patch put to the skin once a week for three weeks, followed by one week off. The patch includes hormones and is up to 99% efficient at preventing pregnancy.
3. **Vaginal ring:** The vaginal ring is a tiny, flexible ring put into the vagina and remains in place for three weeks, followed by one week off. The round includes hormones and is up to 99% efficient at preventing conception.
4. **Depo-Provera injection:** The Depo-Provera injection is a shot that is administered every three months. It includes progestin and is up to 99% efficient at preventing pregnancy.

5. **Hormonal IUD:** The hormonal IUD is a tiny, T-shaped device placed into the uterus and kept in place for three to five years. It produces hormones and is up to 99% efficient in preventing conception.

It's crucial to understand that hormonal birth control methods do not protect against sexually transmitted infections (STIs). Some individuals may have side effects such as headaches, nausea, or mood changes. It's essential to speak to a healthcare practitioner about which type of birth control suits you and to address any concerns or questions you may have.

Combination hormonal contraception (CHC)

Combination hormonal contraception (CHC) is a kind of hormonal birth control comprising estrogen and progestin. This method of contraception is available in numerous forms, including birth control pills, patches, and vaginal rings.

CHC works by inhibiting ovulation, which is the release of an egg from the ovaries. By blocking ovulation, there is no egg accessible for fertilization. Therefore pregnancy cannot occur. In addition to inhibiting ovulation, CHC also thickens cervical mucus, making it more difficult for sperm to access and fertilize an egg. CHC may also thin the uterus lining, making it less susceptible to a fertilized egg.

Following are some of the most prevalent forms of CHC:

1. **Birth control pill:** The birth control pill is a daily medication that includes estrogen and progestin. Many kinds of birth control pills are available, with differing levels of hormones and dose regimens.
2. **Patch:** The birth control patch is a little patch put to the skin once a week for three weeks, followed by one week off. The patch includes both estrogen and progestin.
3. **Vaginal ring:** The vaginal ring is a tiny, flexible ring put into the vagina and remains in place for three weeks, followed by one week off. The crew includes both estrogen and progestin.

CHC successfully prevents pregnancy when taken appropriately, with a failure rate of less than 1% with perfect usage. Nevertheless, it is crucial to remember that CHC does not protect against sexually transmitted infections (STIs), and some individuals may develop adverse effects such as headaches, nausea, or mood changes. It's essential to speak to a healthcare practitioner about which type of birth control suits you and to address any concerns or questions you may have.

Progestin-only contraception

Progestin-only contraception, commonly known as "progestin-only methods" or "mini-pills," is a hormonal birth control that includes just progestin, a synthetic version of the hormone progesterone. These treatments use thickening cervical mucus, making it harder for sperm to access and fertilize an egg. In addition, progestin-only techniques may thin the uterus lining, making it less susceptible to a fertilized egg. Unlike combination hormonal contraception (CHC), progestin-only treatments do not include estrogen.

Below are some of the most frequent kinds of progestin-only contraception:

1. **Progestin-only pill:** The progestin-only pill, often known as the mini-pill, is a daily tablet that contains just progestin. Unlike the combo pill, the mini-pill must be taken simultaneously every day to be effective.
2. **Depo-Provera injection:** The Depo-Provera injection is a shot that is administered every three months. It includes progestin and is up to 99% efficient at preventing pregnancy.
3. **Progestin-only implant:** The progestin-only implant is a short, flexible rod that is put beneath the skin of the upper arm and is effective for up to three years.
4. **Progestin-only IUD:** The progestin-only IUD is a tiny, T-shaped device put into the uterus and may stay in place for up to five years.

Progestin-only techniques may be an excellent solution for people who cannot take estrogen-containing birth control due to medical reasons or personal preferences. But, it's crucial to remember that progestin-only treatments may not be as effective as CHC, and they do not protect against sexually transmitted infections (STIs) (STIs). Moreover, some individuals may develop adverse effects such as irregular bleeding or weight gain. It's essential to speak to a healthcare practitioner about which type of birth control suits you and to address any concerns or questions you may have.

Emergency contraception

Emergency contraception, sometimes known as "the morning-after pill" or "EC," is a method of birth control that may be taken after unprotected intercourse or contraceptive failure to prevent pregnancy. Emergency contraception works by either blocking or delaying ovulation, the release of an egg from the ovary. If ovulation has already happened, emergency contraception cannot prevent conception, but it may still prevent the fertilized egg from implanting in the uterus.

There are numerous methods of emergency contraception available:

1. **Copper Intrauterine Device (IUD):** This is the most effective method of emergency contraception and may be implanted by a healthcare practitioner up to five days following unprotected intercourse or contraceptive failure. The copper IUD may also function as continuing contraception and can stay in place for up to 10 years.
2. **Emergency contraceptive pills (ECPs)** are available in progestin-only and combination hormonal formulations. Progestin-only ECPs are most effective within 72 hours of unprotected sex but can be effective up to five days afterward. Combined hormonal ECPs are most effective within 72 hours of unprotected sex.
3. **Ulipristal acetate (UPA):** This prescription-only emergency contraceptive pill can be effective for up to five days after unprotected sex. UPA works by blocking the hormone progesterone, which is necessary for ovulation.

Emergency contraception is not meant to be used as a regular form of birth control and does not protect against sexually transmitted infections (STIs) (STIs). It's important to talk to a healthcare provider about which method of contraception is suitable for you and to discuss any concerns or questions you may have.

Barrier methods

 Barrier methods are a type of birth control that physically blocks or prevents sperm from reaching an egg. They are called "barrier" methods because they create a barrier between sperm and the cervix, which is the uterine opening. Barrier methods can be used alone or with other types of birth control.

1. Condoms

Condoms are a barrier method of birth control worn over the penis or inserted into the vagina before sex. They are made of either latex, polyurethane, or natural lambskin and work by creating a physical barrier that prevents sperm from entering the vagina and fertilizing an egg.

Condoms effectively prevent pregnancy and sexually transmitted infections (STIs), including HIV. They are commonly accessible and may be bought over the counter at most drugstores, grocery shops, and convenience stores.

There are two primary kinds of condoms: male condoms and female condoms. Male condoms are the most prevalent and are worn over the penis during intercourse. They are available in a range of sizes, textures, and tastes. Female condoms are worn within the vagina and offer protection for both partners.

When worn appropriately and regularly, condoms may be up to 98% effective in preventing pregnancy. It's crucial to use a fresh condom for each act of intercourse, to follow the directions on the container, and to inspect for any damage before using. Condoms may be used alone or with other birth control methods for increased protection.

Furthermore to avoiding pregnancy and STIs, condoms offer various additional advantages. They are non-hormonal, meaning they do not impact the body's normal hormone levels and have no adverse effects. They are also straightforward and do not require a prescription or a healthcare provider's visit.

2. Diaphragms

A diaphragm is a sort of barrier technique of birth control that is a soft, dome-shaped device made of silicone or latex that is put into the vagina and positioned over the cervix to prevent sperm from entering the uterus. It works by producing a barrier that inhibits the sperm from accessing the egg and fertilizing it. Diaphragms are reusable and may be cleaned and used again.

A healthcare expert fits diaphragms to guarantee each person's optimum size and form. They may be used with spermicide, which destroys sperm, for further protection against pregnancy. Spermicide is often administered to the diaphragm before insertion, and it helps to immobilize or kill sperm that may come into contact with it.

Diaphragms may successfully prevent pregnancy when worn appropriately and regularly. Still, their efficiency can vary depending on several variables, such as the type of spermicide used, the fit of the diaphragm, and how frequently it is used.

Some possible advantages of diaphragms are that they are non-hormonal and do not have the potential adverse effects of hormonal birth control techniques. They also offer protection against sexually transmitted infections (STIs) that can be transmitted through genital contact.

However, there are also some potential drawbacks to using diaphragms. They require insertion and removal, which can be inconvenient for some people. They may also be less successful than other kinds of birth control, such as hormonal techniques or intrauterine devices (IUDs) (IUDs). Moreover, diaphragms might raise the risk of urinary tract infections (UTIs) in certain persons.

Diaphragms might be a helpful alternative for those searching for non-hormonal, non-invasive birth control that they can handle themselves. It's vital to speak to a healthcare practitioner to explore if a diaphragm is the proper form of birth control for you and to learn how to use it correctly.

3. Cervical caps

A cervical cap is a sort of barrier technique of birth control that is a tiny, flexible cup made of silicone or latex put into the vagina and positioned over the cervix to prevent sperm from entering the uterus. It works by producing a barrier that inhibits the sperm from accessing the egg and fertilizing it.

Cervical caps exist in various sizes and must be fitted by a healthcare expert to guarantee each person's optimum size and form. They are supposed to be used with spermicide, a chemical that destroys sperm, for further protection against pregnancy. Spermicide is often put on the cervical cap before insertion, which helps to immobilize or kill sperm that may come into contact with it.

Cervical caps can be effective at preventing pregnancy when used correctly and consistently. Still, their effectiveness can vary depending on various factors, such as the type of spermicide used, the fit of the cap, and how consistently it is used.

Some potential benefits of cervical caps include the fact that they are non-hormonal and do not have the possible side effects of hormonal birth control methods. They are also reusable and may be cleaned and used again.

Yet, there are also some possible downsides to utilizing cervical caps. They need insertion and removal, which might be bothersome for specific individuals. They may also be less successful than other kinds of birth control, such as hormonal techniques or intrauterine devices (IUDs). Moreover, cervical caps might raise the risk of urinary tract infections (UTIs) in certain patients.

Cervical caps can be a good option for people looking for non-hormonal, non-invasive birth control that they can control themselves. It's important to talk to a healthcare provider to discuss whether a cervical cap is a suitable method of birth control for you and to learn how to use it correctly.

4. Spermicides

Spermicides are a contraceptive method that contains chemicals that immobilize or kill sperm. They come in various forms, including gels, foams, creams, suppositories, and films, and are inserted into the vagina before sexual intercourse to prevent sperm from reaching the egg.

Spermicides create a chemical barrier that prevents sperm from moving through the cervix and reaching the egg. They often include a substance called nonoxynol-9, which is the active element that immobilizes or kills the sperm.

Spermicides may be used alone or in conjunction with other barrier methods of birth control, such as condoms, diaphragms, and cervical caps. When used alone, spermicides have a greater failure rate than other birth control methods, such as hormonal techniques or intrauterine devices (IUDs) (IUDs). But, when used with another barrier strategy, they may further protect against pregnancy.

Some possible advantages of spermicides are that they are non-hormonal and do not have the potential adverse effects of hormonal birth control techniques. They are also accessible without a prescription and are uncomplicated to use.

Yet, there are also some possible downsides to utilizing spermicides. They need implantation into the vagina, which might be difficult for some individuals. They may also cause discomfort or allergic responses in certain people. Moreover, spermicides are less efficient in preventing conception than other types of birth control.

Spermicides may be a helpful alternative for those searching for non-hormonal, non-invasive birth control that they can handle themselves. It's important to talk to a healthcare provider to discuss whether spermicides are a suitable method of birth control for you and to learn how to use them correctly.

Long-acting reversible contraception (LARC)

Long-acting reversible contraception (LARC) is a category of birth control methods that offer highly effective and long-lasting protection against pregnancy. LARC methods include intrauterine devices (IUDs) and contraceptive implants.

1. Intrauterine devices (IUDs)

Intrauterine devices (IUDs) are tiny, T-shaped devices that are put into the uterus by a healthcare professional as a type of long-acting reversible contraception (LARC) (LARC). There are two kinds of IUDs: copper and hormonal.

Copper IUDs are wrapped in copper wire and act by causing an inflammatory response that hinders fertilization and implantation of the fertilized egg. They may stay effective for up to 10 years and are a suitable alternative for persons who cannot use hormonal birth control methods.

Hormonal IUDs produce a tiny amount of progestin, which thickens cervical mucus and thins the lining of the uterus, making it difficult for sperm to access and fertilize an egg. Hormonal IUDs can remain effective for 3-5 years, depending on the specific type.

IUDs are highly effective at preventing pregnancy, with a failure rate of less than 1%. They are also a low-maintenance form of birth control, as they require no daily action by the user. Once inserted, IUDs can remain in place for several years, depending on the type.

Some potential benefits of IUDs include that they are highly effective, long-lasting, and do not require daily action by the user. They also do not interfere with sexual activity, and fertility returns quickly once the device is removed.

However, there are also some potential drawbacks to using IUDs. They require insertion by a healthcare provider, which can be a barrier to access for some people. They can also cause side effects such as irregular bleeding or cramping; some people may not like the idea of implanted devices in their bodies.

IUDs can be a good option for people who want highly effective, long-lasting birth control that they do not have to think about daily. It's important to talk to a healthcare provider to discuss whether an IUD is the correct method of birth control for you and to learn about the potential benefits and drawbacks.

2. Implants

Contraceptive implants are short, flexible rods implanted beneath the upper arm's skin by a healthcare professional as a method of long-acting reversible contraception (LARC) (LARC). They produce a continuous dosage of progestin, which thickens cervical mucus and thins the uterus lining, making it difficult for sperm to access and fertilize an egg.

Implants successfully prevent pregnancy, with a failure rate of less than 1%. Depending on the precise variety, they may stay effective for up to 3 years. After being implanted, implants need no daily activity by the user.

Some possible advantages of implants are that they are very effective, long-lasting, and do not need daily activity by the user. They also do not interfere with sexual activity, and fertility recovers fast after the device is withdrawn.

Yet, there are also some possible downsides to utilizing implants. They need insertion by a healthcare practitioner, which might be a barrier to access for specific individuals. They may also bring adverse effects such as irregular bleeding or mood problems, and some individuals may not enjoy having a device implanted in their bodies.

Sterilization

Sterilization is a permanent kind of birth control that includes a surgical or non-surgical treatment to halt the release of eggs or sperm, therefore preventing pregnancy

Female sterilization (tubal ligation)

Female sterilization, commonly known as tubal ligation, is a surgical operation to permanently prevent conception. It includes restricting or closing the fallopian tubes, which are the tubes that transfer eggs from the ovaries to the uterus. By doing so, the egg cannot be fertilized by sperm, and pregnancy cannot ensue.

Various other ways may be used to conduct tubal ligation, but the most frequent approach is laparoscopic. During this surgery, tiny incisions are created in the belly, and a laparoscope (a thin, illuminated tube) is introduced into one of the incisions. The surgeon uses the laparoscope to see the fallopian lines, then implants little clips or rings to block them.

Tubal ligation may also be done using a mini-laparotomy, which entails making a tiny incision in the lower abdomen and using a small instrument to seal or block the fallopian tubes. Another approach is hysteroscopy sterilization, which involves putting a remote device through the cervix and into the uterus to stop the fallopian lines.

Tubal ligation is a very successful birth control technique, with a failure rate of less than 1%. Nevertheless, it is a permanent form of birth control and should only be explored by those who are positive they do not want to have children in the future. Although the treatment may occasionally be reversed, it is not usually effective.

Some possible dangers and problems of tubal ligation include bleeding, infection, harm to other organs, and surgery failure. Healing time might vary depending on the precise technique, but most women can return to their typical activities within a few days to a week following the surgery.

Male sterilization (vasectomy)

Male sterilization, often known as vasectomy, is a surgical operation to permanently prevent conception. It includes cutting or obstructing the vas deferens, the tubes that deliver sperm from the testicles to the urethra. By doing so, the semen that is ejaculated during sexual intercourse does not contain sperm, and pregnancy cannot occur.

A tiny incision is performed in the scrotum during a vasectomy, and the vas deferens are cut, tied, or blocked. The treatment is usually done under local anesthesia and takes 20–30 minutes. Following the surgery, men are often recommended to relax for a day or two and to avoid heavy exercise for a few days.

Vasectomy is a very successful form of birth control, with a failure rate of less than 1%. Nevertheless, it is a permanent form of birth control and should only be explored by those who are positive they do not want to have children in the future. Although the treatment may occasionally be reversed, it is not usually effective.

Some possible dangers and consequences of vasectomy include bleeding, infection, pain or discomfort in the testicles, and failure of the treatment. Nonetheless, the risks associated with vasectomy are typically believed to be negligible.

It's crucial to remember that vasectomy does not protect against sexually transmitted infections (STIs). Thus it is still vital to use condoms or other types of protection to avoid STIs.

A vasectomy might be a suitable choice for men who are confident they do not want to have children in the future and are searching for a permanent type of birth control. It's vital to speak to a healthcare practitioner to explore if vasectomy is the correct type of birth control for you and to learn about the possible advantages and cons.

CHAPTER 3

How to Select a Birth Control Method

Selecting a birth control technique that works best for you may be a personal choice, and there are many aspects to consider. Here are some factors to consider while selecting a birth control method:

1. **Effectiveness:** How efficient is the approach in preventing pregnancy? Some ways are more effective, so determine the protection you need.

2. **Health:** Certain procedures may not be suited for everyone. It's crucial to speak to a healthcare practitioner about any health issues or concerns you may have and any drugs you're taking to establish which procedures may be safe for you.

3. **Convenience:** How simple is the approach to use? Some techniques demand more work than others, such as taking a pill simultaneously every day, while others are more low-maintenance, like an IUD that may remain in place for many years.

4. **Cost:** Certain techniques may be more costly than others, so examining the financial component of birth control is vital.

5. **Side effects:** Every treatment has possible side effects, so it's vital to speak to a healthcare practitioner about any concerns and be informed of the potential dangers connected with each approach.

6. **STI protection:** Certain techniques, such as condoms, may also give protection against sexually transmitted diseases (STIs), while others do not. If STI protection is essential to you, choose a method that provides it.

Ultimately, the ideal form of birth control is the one you feel most comfortable taking regularly. Talking to a healthcare expert will help you evaluate which strategy may be suitable for you, depending on your unique requirements and preferences.

7. **Plans:** If you hope to have children shortly, you may want to pick a procedure that is readily reversible or doesn't impair your fertility in the long run.

Personal preferences

Personal tastes are an essential thing to consider when selecting a birth control technique. Every person is different, and what works well for one person may not work well for another. Here are some personal preferences to keep in mind when selecting a method:

Hormonal vs. non-hormonal: Some individuals choose not to utilize hormonal techniques, while others may prefer them since they may help regulate menstrual cycles and alleviate symptoms of PMS.

1. **Long-acting vs. short-acting:** Some individuals may choose a technique that must only be used periodically. Others may prefer a method that gives long-lasting protection without regular intervention.
2. **Daily versus periodic:** Certain treatments, like the pill or patch, need daily or near-daily usage, while others, like the shot or IUD, only need to be delivered occasionally.
3. **Partner participation:** Certain methods, like condoms, need partner involvement, while others, like the implant or IUD, may be used without your spouse having to do anything.
4. **Reversibility:** If you're not sure if you want to have children in the future or if you want to have them soon, you may want to pick a readily reversible procedure.

Ultimately, selecting a strategy that you are comfortable with and that matches your lifestyle and interests is crucial. Talking to a healthcare expert will help you better understand your choices and decide which technique will work best for you.

Medical considerations

When selecting a birth control technique, medical concerns are an essential issue to bear in mind. These are some medical considerations to consider:

1. **Health problems:** Some health issues or drugs may impair the safety or efficacy of various birth control techniques. For example, women with a history of blood clots may be unable to utilize hormonal techniques since they might raise the risk of blood clots.
2. **Age:** Various strategies may be more or less acceptable depending on a person's age. For example, older women may be better suited for non-hormonal treatments, whereas younger women may prefer hormonal ones.
3. **Family history:** Some health disorders, such as breast cancer or heart disease, may run in families. If you have a family history of these disorders, evaluating how specific birth control methods may increase your risk is crucial.
4. **Fertility goals:** If you wish to have children in the future, you may want to pick a readily reversible treatment that doesn't damage your long-term fertility.
5. **Allergies:** Some individuals may be allergic to particular kinds of birth control, such as latex condoms or some types of spermicide.
6. **Side effects:** All birth control methods have possible side effects, so it's vital to understand what they are and how they can impact you.

Speaking to a healthcare practitioner about any medical issues or drugs you're taking is crucial to deciding which approaches may be safe and beneficial for you. They can help you assess the advantages and hazards of numerous alternatives and decide which method is best for your unique circumstances.

Effectiveness ratings

Efficacy rates are a vital consideration when selecting a birth control treatment. The efficacy of a technique relates to its capacity to prevent pregnancy when performed appropriately and regularly. Following are some typical efficacy rates for various forms of birth control:

1. **Hormonal techniques:** Combination hormonal contraceptives (such as the pill, patch, and ring) and progestin-only treatments (such as the shot and implant) are very successful, with a failure rate of less than 1% when used appropriately.

2. **Barrier techniques:** Condoms, diaphragms, and cervical caps are less successful than hormonal approaches, with failure rates ranging from 12-24% with the usual usage.

3. **Long-acting reversible contraception (LARC):** Intrauterine devices (IUDs) and implants are the most successful techniques available, with less than 1% failure rates when used appropriately.

4. **Sterilization:** Female sterilization (tubal ligation) and male sterilization (vasectomy) are very successful, with less than 1% failure rates.

It's vital to bear in mind that no form of birth control is 100% successful, and the efficiency of a technique might vary depending on how frequently and accurately it is used. While picking a method, it's crucial to evaluate your specific circumstances and choose a way that you are comfortable with and that matches your lifestyle and interests. Talking to a healthcare expert will help you better understand your choices and decide which technique will work best for you.

CHAPTER 4

How to Use Birth Control

The method of birth control you choose will impact how you utilize it. These are some basic instructions for using some of the most prevalent types of birth control:

1. **Hormonal methods:** Birth control pills, patches, and vaginal rings are typically taken for 21 to 28 days per cycle, followed by a 7-day respite during which you may have your monthly period. Progestin-only techniques, such as the shot and the implant, need periodic injections or insertions.

2. **Barrier methods:** Condoms are used by putting them over the penis before sexual activity. Diaphragms and cervical caps are put into the vagina before sexual activity and need spermicide to be successful.

3. **Long-acting reversible contraception (LARC):** A healthcare professional implants IUDs and implants and may offer long-term contraception for many years.

4. **Sterilization:** Female sterilization (tubal ligation) and male sterilization (vasectomy) involve surgery and should be regarded as permanent measures of reproductive control.

No matter the type of birth control you pick, using it regularly and appropriately to optimize its efficacy is crucial. Be sure to read the directions carefully and consult your healthcare practitioner if you have any questions or concerns about how to use your chosen type of birth control. Also, it's vital to continue taking birth control until you are ready to get pregnant and to utilize barrier techniques, such as condoms, to protect against sexually transmitted illnesses.

Instructions for usage of various approaches

Hormonal methods: Birth control pills, patches, and vaginal rings should be used according to the recommendations supplied by your healthcare professional or the manufacturer. Generally, you will take or utilize them every day simultaneously, including throughout your menstrual cycle. Progestin-only procedures, such as the shot and the implant, need periodic injections or insertions from a healthcare professional.

Barrier methods: Condoms should be used every time you have intercourse, from start to end. To use a condom, pull it from the box and unroll it over the erect penis, squeezing the tip to provide room for semen. Following ejaculation, grip the base of the condom and slowly draw it out to prevent leaking any semen. Diaphragms and cervical caps are put into the vagina before sexual activity and need spermicide to be successful. They should be kept in place for at least 6 hours after intercourse and removed within 24 hours.

Long-acting reversible contraception (LARC): A healthcare professional implants IUDs and implants and may offer long-term contraception for many years. Depending on the variety, IUDs may be kept in place for 3–10 years, whereas implants can be effective for up to 3 years. Your healthcare practitioner will offer advice on how to check the location of your IUD or implant and when to get it removed or replaced.

Sterilization: Female sterilization (tubal ligation) and male sterilization (vasectomy) involve surgery and should be regarded as permanent measures of reproductive control. Your healthcare practitioner will advise on preparing for the operation and what to anticipate during and after the surgery.

It's crucial to use your chosen form of birth control regularly and appropriately to enhance its efficacy. Be sure to read the directions carefully and consult your healthcare practitioner if you have any questions or concerns about how to use your chosen type of birth control.

Common side effects and how to control them

Various methods of birth control may have distinct side effects; some individuals may have adverse effects while others do not. These are some frequent adverse effects of multiple types of birth control and how to handle them:

Hormonal methods: Birth control pills, patches, and vaginal rings may produce adverse effects such as nausea, headaches, mood changes, and changes in monthly flow. To manage these side effects, you can try taking your pill or using your patch or ring at a different time of day, taking it with food, or switching to another method of birth control. Progestin-only methods such as the shot and the implant may cause irregular bleeding, weight gain, and mood changes. Some side effects may improve with time or with a change in dose.

Barrier methods: Condoms may cause irritation or allergic responses, especially if you or your partner has a latex allergy. To handle these adverse effects, you might consider switching to non-latex condoms or using a suitable lubricant for your skin. Diaphragms and cervical caps may cause pain or vaginal irritation. To control these adverse effects, use water-based lubrication and avoid keeping the device longer than suggested.

Long-acting reversible contraception (LARC): IUDs and implants may cause irregular bleeding, cramping, or pain during implantation. These side effects may improve with time, but you may manage them by using over-the-counter pain medicines or a heating pad. If you have severe discomfort or significant bleeding, call your healthcare professional.

Sterilization: Female and male sterilization are typically well-tolerated and do not produce significant adverse effects. But, like with any operation, there is a risk of infection, bleeding, or other consequences. Follow your healthcare provider's recommendations for preparing for and recuperating from the process.

If you experience side effects that are persistent or severe, or if you have concerns about how your chosen method of birth control is affecting your health, talk to your healthcare provider. They can help you evaluate the benefits and risks of different techniques and suggest alternative options if necessary.

How to handle missed doses or failed contraception

Handling missed doses or failed contraception depends on the birth control method you use. Here are some general guidelines:

1. **Hormonal methods:** If you miss a pill, patch, or ring, check the instructions that came with your birth control to determine what to do. Depending on how many doses you have missed and when you are in your cycle, you may need to use backup contraception (such as condoms) for a set length or take emergency contraception if you have had unprotected sex. If you suffer vomiting or diarrhea within a few hours of taking your pill, patch, or ring, you may also need to take backup contraception.

2. **Barrier methods**: If a condom breaks or comes off during sex, you may need emergency contraception to lower your chance of pregnancy. If you have used a diaphragm or cervical cap and are afraid that it may have migrated out of place, you may verify its position and apply a backup technique (such as spermicide) if required.

3. **Long-acting reversible contraception (LARC):** If you are using an IUD or implant and are worried that it may have moved or been dislodged, you may check its position or ask your healthcare professional to do so. If you have had unprotected sex after the device has changed or if it has been longer than the suggested period following implantation, you may need to take emergency contraception.

4. **Sterilization:** If you have undergone female or male sterilization and are worried it may have failed, speak to your healthcare physician about your alternatives. Although the failure rate for sterilization treatments is minimal, it is possible for the surgery to reverse itself or for the fallopian tubes to grow back together.

If you have had unprotected sex or are worried about the efficacy of your chosen method of birth control, speak to your healthcare professional about your alternatives. They can help you estimate your risk of pregnancy and propose different ways or backup contraception if required.

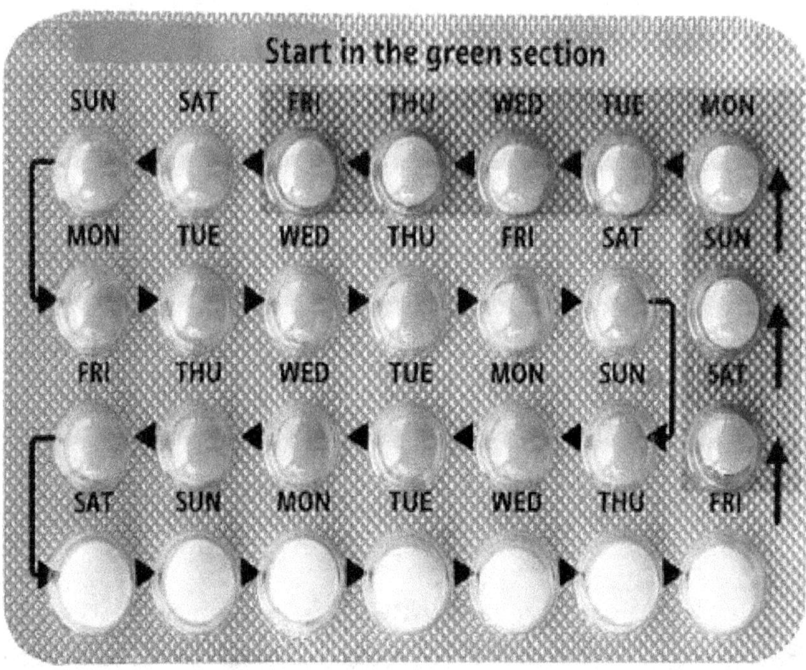

CONCLUSION

Birth control is essential for preventing unintended pregnancies and improving reproductive health. With a wide range of options, individuals can choose a method that best fits their needs and lifestyle. It is essential to consider factors such as personal preferences, medical considerations, and effectiveness rates when selecting a plan and to use the method correctly and consistently to maximize its benefits. It is also essential to discuss any concerns or questions with a healthcare provider and stay informed about new developments and advancements in birth control options. Overall, birth control empowers individuals to take control of their reproductive health and make informed decisions about their bodies and futures.

Some important points about birth control:

Birth control is any method or device used to prevent unintended pregnancy.

There are many types of birth control, including hormonal methods, barrier methods, long-acting reversible contraception, and sterilization.

1. Hormonal birth control methods include combined hormonal contraception (CHC) and progestin-only contraception, which work by preventing ovulation.
2. Barrier birth control methods, such as condoms, diaphragms, and cervical caps, physically block sperm from reaching the egg.
3. Long-acting reversible contraception (LARC) includes methods such as intrauterine devices (IUDs) and implants, which are highly effective and require less maintenance than other methods.
4. Sterilization, including tubal ligation for women and vasectomy for men, is a permanent form of birth control.

When choosing a birth control method, one must consider personal preferences, medical considerations, and effectiveness rates. Using birth control consistently and correctly is essential to maximize its effectiveness and prevent unintended pregnancy.

Different birth control methods' side effects vary, and discussing any concerns with a healthcare provider is essential. Male birth control options are limited, and each has potential side effects.

Birth control is an essential tool for improving reproductive health and preventing unintended pregnancies. Individuals should work with healthcare providers to choose the best method for their needs and lifestyle.

If you are considering using birth control, speaking to a healthcare provider who can help you choose the best option for your needs and provide guidance on how to use it effectively is essential. Your healthcare provider can also help you manage any side effects or issues that may arise while using birth control.

Don't be frightened or ashamed to discuss the matter with your healthcare professional. They can help you make educated choices regarding your reproductive health. Remember that selecting a birth control technique is a personal choice, and what works for one person may not be the best match for another. Your healthcare provider can provide information and resources to help you make the right choice.

Taking control of your reproductive health by using birth control is a responsible and empowering decision. By speaking to a healthcare provider, you can ensure that you are making informed decisions about your body and taking the necessary steps to prevent unintended pregnancy.